Anna Mancini

I0104422

Depression And How Your Dreams Can Help You Avoid It

What Depression Is, and How Its Earliest Signs Appear
in Your Dreams While There Is Still Time to Avoid It

Buenos Books America
www.buenosbooks.us

ISBN: 978-1-963580-01-3

Imprint: Buenos Books America LLC
www.buenosbooks.us

WARNING:

This is not a medical book; I am not a doctor and I offer no treatments. My aim is to share my experience in the field of dreams. The aim of this book is to help readers manage their life-energy better with the help of their dreams and it explains how to avoid falling into depressive states caused by lack of energy in the body.

This book is not for those unfortunate souls who are already so depressed that they have to take drugs. They should persevere with their usual doctors and conventional treatments, which, in suppressing dreams, make it impossible by the same token to make use of the therapeutic power of dreams. I regret to say this, and if you have the desire, the opportunity, and the strength, try to get medical help to free yourself from drugs and regain your natural zest for life and your dream abilities. If you decide to take such a path, reading this book can help you better understand why you have fallen into depression and how you can use this understanding to cooperate better with your caregivers.

INTRODUCTION

Careful observation of our dreams and their links with reality increases the awareness of the energetic dimension of the human body. Without this energy flowing in our bodies, none of us would be alive. Such observation gradually unveils the natural laws of the functioning of human energy. In the long run, failure to conform to these laws, even out of pure ignorance, leads to lack of energy, which in turn triggers most depressive states or physical illnesses.

Chinese acupuncturists are familiar with the "intangible anatomy" of human beings, and they achieve remarkable results by acting directly on it with their needles. According to ancient Chinese medicine, human beings are part of a broader natural system influencing their health and vitality, and they have to continually make exchanges with their natural environment to stay alive. Ancient Chinese acupuncture charts show that the meridians of energy within the human body are influenced by cosmic energies.

Indian yogis are mostly focused on increasing their energy in order to reach states of consciousness and develop faculties which most Westerners cannot even imagine. They have invented many techniques for this purpose. Instead, most Westerners pay little attention to this aspect of life and tend to hover constantly at the lowest point of the energy scale, that is to say where there is insufficient energy to allow joyful life and psychological well-being.

Yet there was a time when the West was more aware of this energetic dimension of human life, and some evidence can be found in legends or, for example, in the iconography of the Catholic church, which has often depicted the energy that emanates from the saints as light flowing from their hands or hearts, or as haloes around their heads.

Human life-energy was also central to the ancient Egyptian civilization, as evidenced by ancient Egyptian texts and artifacts. Ancient Egyptian priests were mostly interested in the functioning of the laws of LIFE. It is no mere coincidence that the symbol of life, namely the

Ankh cross, is omnipresent in their texts and images. In some wall paintings, we can see small Ankh crosses presented to the mouth of the Pharaoh by tiny hands placed at the end of the sun's rays. All the Egyptian gods and goddesses are givers of life. This is symbolized by them standing with the ankh cross in their hands, or squatting with it on their knees. The goddess Maat is the personification of life, which circulates in the cosmos, feeds the sun, and animates all living beings "down to the smallest worm," as was clearly stated by ancient Egyptian texts.

We are all penetrated by a current of life, with its intensity and tonality varying according to many factors, for example, our personality, nationality, heredity, state of mind, lifestyle, environment, and eating habits.

The human body is not only about matter and chemistry; it is also about energy. Modern science has put the material and chemical aspect of the body at the top of its agenda and has almost excised energy from its investigations. Yet, as the correct flow of energy in the body is essential for maintaining good health, our

—

Western civilization is paying dearly for not taking sufficient account of the energy dimension of human life. Focused on material wealth and money, so-called developed countries have not succeeded in making their people happy and healthy, physically and mentally. Instead, they have created hordes of depressed, sleepless, drugged, sick, unhappy people who are also undermined by all kinds of addictions and are functioning "in slow motion" physically, intellectually, and emotionally, to such an extent that living in such miserable conditions no longer interests some individuals and they prefer to take their own lives. For example, of the European countries, France has, unfortunately, the highest suicide rate. According to its statisticians, the "factor most associated with suicidal thoughts is the fact of having experienced a depressive episode during the year." I dare not imagine what would happen in this country if suddenly all its sleepless, depressed, distressed, or "tortured" inhabitants no longer had access to their usual drugs. French people are, in fact, the world's largest consumers of psychiatric drugs; one in four uses them regularly, and this has strongly increased with the COVID pandemic.

The increasing number of depressed people in this country generates a sad atmosphere that is not a pleasant environment for others. It is a pity, since this situation could be perfectly well avoided.

Western medicine attributes the cause of depression to various determining factors, such as a traumatic childhood or health problems that have triggered a great loss of vitality. But science focused on the study of material realities has not yet developed the tools necessary to observe the laws of life, which are, instead, immaterial. As a result, we are particularly powerless to help patients make up for their "lack of life" and regain their natural zest. The drugs we give to the mentally ill are only "crutches" to help them endure the sad consequences of lack of vitality in the body. They do not cure depression, and they have horrible side effects, like dependency and loss of the ability to dream.

In this book, I would like to share my experience and shed a different, more joyful, more optimistic light on this aspect of the human condition. I have observed for more than thirty years the functioning of the human body at the junction between dream and reality, and I have conducted experiments that are impossible to carry out in laboratories because they presuppose observing realities that are beyond the scope of modern science and applying the adage "know yourself." A deep intimate self-observation of our functioning at the junction between dream and reality is the best way to understand all the aspects of life that lie beyond the current fields of scientific investigation.

The conscious mind, as well as those of scientists, is primarily focused on material life and the outside world. On the contrary, the number one goal of the subconscious mind and the body is the preservation of LIFE. Therefore, they never fail to inform us about everything that is harming and decreasing it. They keep us informed mainly through dreams but also through certain physical signals. Dreams always sound the alarm bell when we are losing too much energy and in danger of falling into a depressive state. They often offer a solution long before it is too late to avoid depression.

By observing your dreams, you will be able to get to know yourself better, both psychologically and physically. You will be able to better manage your energy and avoid wasting or losing it through ignorance. You will be able to understand how to make smarter life choices from an energy standpoint, which will allow you to always have enough energy at your disposal to stay mentally healthy and to enjoy your life. Why always give priority to material life? What good is all the wealth in the world if we have lost the drive to live and are struggling with depression?

I am now going to discuss the main activities in which we tend to lose significant amounts of energy. Then, I will explain what we can do to gain energy. This information will be useful in allowing you to make the most of your dreams by observing through them how you, personally, gain or lose energy in these activities. The same activity can increase or decrease energy, depending on the individual, how it is performed, or where it takes place. When it comes to managing your life-energy, dreams are such a valuable feedback tool. So, learn how to use them!

After examining the most common areas of loss and gain of vital energy, we will consider examples of dreams that signal damage to our energy, which after a while, should nothing be done to remedy the situation, may trigger a depression. We will conclude this book by opening new horizons through the presentation of some little known, forgotten, or once forbidden means, destined to recharge the human body with energy and therefore address the lack of energy in the body which is the main cause of depression.

CHAPTER 1: How we tend to lose our energy

In this chapter, I will discuss the most common ways we humans have become accustomed to losing our energy. This does not mean that we should stop doing the things which cost us significant energy; we just need to go about them in a smarter way and learn how to harvest enough energy before we expend it on "energetically expensive" activities. I will not discuss in this book the spiritual (generally speaking, that is to say, non-religious) aspects of loss of energy, which are too complex for most people with no experience of their dream world; this will be addressed in another book or video. I invite you to subscribe to my YouTube channel so that you will be notified when I post a new video.[1]

The most common causes of energy loss are:

-1) Digestion and diet

---

[1] *https://www.YouTube.com/c/LaSignificationdesRevesAutrement*

-2) Sexuality

-3) The material environment

-4) The human environment

-5) Negative thoughts

-6) Too much or unsuitable work and sport.

Note that in these activities, many people consume too much energy, while some gain energy because they have learned to manage it better, and you can do the same. Read the following information and observe your dreams, and you will be able to better manage these energy-draining activities and even turn them into recharging ones.

1) The digestive system: food, digestion, and elimination

Have you ever heard of "breatharians"? Breatharians manage to live by "eating" only solar energy. Jasmuheen, an Australian woman, has been very active in circulating information about breatharianism in the West. She has received much criticism and disbelief, yet feeding on solar energy is nothing new: Indian yogis have been doing it for millennia. To feed directly on "solar energy," zero energy expense is necessary for digestion. This is very interesting because we have to expend considerable energy through digestion to extract life-energy from the food we eat.

Breatharians, who expend almost nothing on "digestion," always win in terms of energy when they feed themselves and therefore end up increasing their vital energy through their "food." Unfortunately, this is not always the case for us, as we will see later. But there is hope, at least, for the future, since according to some spiritual masters, when humanity is more spiritually developed, we will all feed directly on light, like the few people in the world who can do so now without dying. However, neither you nor I have yet reached this point! Since we are forced to ingest food and digest it to stay alive, we would do well to take an interest in the digestive process to make better use of it from an energy point of view.

Digestion is a highly complex, multidimensional phenomenon which mainly consists in extracting life from matter. To digest, we use matter (food, digestive juices), air (breathing), and energy (the "fire" of digestion). The emotions we have during and around our meals affect our digestion and can even block it if they cause too much stress.

Nutrition goes far beyond a simple matter of intake of minerals, vitamins, fats, or carbohydrates, and their chemical transformation in the stomach; it also has an equally important energetic aspect. Foods also contain energy. Fruits and vegetables, for example, are loaded with solar energy, and when we digest them, like the breatharians, we feed on solar energy, but we do so through the medium of food instead of directly from our environment.

Through personal study of your dreams, you will see for yourself how your digestion functions from an energetic and also material point of view. You will see more clearly through your dreams how the different foods you eat are affecting your energy positively or negatively. In this regard, you can make lots of experiments with foods by introducing or removing certain foods from your diet and observing what occurs in your dreams. You will find that some foods recharge you considerably, while other foods considered healthy are not suitable for you and instead decrease your vitality. You may find that other foods give you very little energy because you have to expend too much energy to digest them. I'll give you some personal examples to illustrate this:

Orange juice:

Orange juice is known to be good for the health, especially for the high level of vitamin C it contains. I began to notice that every time I drank it, I dreamed that I had swallowed a glass of acid.

I didn't realize right away that orange juice wasn't good for me. I really like its odor and taste, but thanks to my dreams, I came to realize that it would be better to avoid drinking it because it was harming my body and also messing with my digestion.

Honey:

One winter in Paris, after a few weeks without sun, I bought some excellent quality Greek honey and took great delight in wolfing some down before going to sleep. The next night, my dreams had more vivid colors and were full of light. They unfolded peacefully in beautiful, sunny, natural landscapes. I deduced from these dreams that I had benefited from the high-energy charge and special vibration of this honey.

I later observed that this phenomenon did not occur with all types of honey, nor did it occur in summer. At this time of the year, consuming honey has a weaker impact in terms of energy because my life-energy is higher than during the long gray Parisian winters.

Sometimes, you won't even need your dreams to become aware of the effect of certain foods! Your stomach, belly, and post-meal mood will tell you how you should eat to increase your vitality instead of decreasing it.

There is no ideal diet that works for everyone. Each of us is different, and we must learn to select foods we can digest easily and which in turn give us plenty of energy. By observing your dreams, you will uncover useful information for making better food choices so that they help you increase your vitality instead of the opposite. Of course, you can also make smart use of your dream faculties to figure out how to lose or gain weight.

Nowadays, food which should normally bring us a lot of energy instead brings little or even decreases it, to the point of being, for some, a trigger of depression. This is then "cured" with antidepressants, which negatively impact digestion. Let's see why.

1.1 Why do we lose too much energy nowadays by feeding ourselves?

a) A diet that contains little life

We all know that our modern foods have become "denatured" and contain little life-energy. However, we still need to expend a lot of energy to digest them.

Therefore, contrary to the foods of the past, which were full of life and usually increased our vitality once digested, our modern food brings us, at best, much less energy. Unfortunately, in many cases, it can even cause an energy deficit and contribute over the years to gradual general decline in the body's vitality. Allied with other factors, such decline of energy can lead at some point to the onset of depression. Fortunately, it is quite easy to remedy this problem by making better alimentary choices. Generally, it is enough to opt for a diet with more fruit and vegetables, as fresh and natural as possible, and to exclude denatured and dead industrial foods, which we often ingest only to our detriment.

b) Disorders of the digestive system due to the presence of parasites

In the past, people regularly dewormed themselves because they knew it was necessary to stay healthy. Nowadays, it is widely accepted that cats, dogs, horses, and small children need to be regularly dewormed, but adults generally think they are free from parasites. However, if they paid attention to their dreams, they could detect the presence of parasites in their digestive tract and do what they absolutely should in that case: eliminate them right away. If there is one thing that consumes the energy of humans and depresses them, it is the presence of parasites in the digestive tract, and especially worms in the small intestine.

Why do parasites deplete our energy? It is very simple: while a person hosting parasites expends a lot of energy digesting food, she receives little from the digested food because the parasites located in the most favorable position—that is, right at the exit of the stomach—enjoy the fruits of digestion, and, moreover, they discharge their metabolic waste into their host. It is so striking that the symptoms of depression listed by modern medicine are so akin to the symptoms of the presence of parasites in the digestive tract. I invite you to do your own research in this area, as I am not a doctor and therefore cannot give you medical advice on how to get rid of parasites. You will greatly benefit from reading Hulda Clark's book *The Cure of All Diseases*.

Simply eliminating parasites from the digestive tract can at times be enough to cure depression and suddenly bring back the zest for life. Today, many people are simply depressed because the many parasites they host prevent them from getting enough energy through eating. Fortunately, depression doesn't ensue right after a parasite infestation; it takes some time and if we use our dreams to learn to detect as early as possible their presence in our body, we can take immediate action and avoid lots of inconveniences. Sometimes, infected people have no other symptoms than fatigue and depression, and therefore neither they nor their doctors think about eliminating parasites from the body. Instead, in cases of chronic fatigue, many people take more vitamins and minerals, and make their parasites even happier.

It is easy to get rid of most parasites, which may also cause bloating and other digestive disorders, nervousness, and even insomnia. The faster you act, the less energy you lose to parasites. Observing your dreams is very useful in this area because through clear or symbolic dreams, the body almost always signals the presence of parasites. I will now give you some examples of such dreams.

People trained in the art of dreaming can use their dreams to see clearly inside their bodies and organs, and check if they are hosting parasites. They can identify them clearly and even see their eggs and inside the eggs, or see the eggs enlarged as if under a sophisticated, powerful microscope. Shamans and some people under hypnosis also have the ability to see clearly what is happening within the human body.

But do not worry if you are not yet able to achieve this clear perception in your dreams, because you will otherwise get this information through common dreams that warn you of parasites. Let's see some examples. (Obviously, every person is different and personal dream observation work is necessary to fully understand one's personal dream language.)

<u>Examples of dreams that signal the presence of parasites</u>
<u>in the digestive tract:</u>

You regularly dream that strangers are squatting in your kitchen; you see them under the table, in the cupboards, and they ignore you when you ask them to leave. You also realize that they have been living there for a long time, and that all this time, you had never been less than aware of their presence, and you feel that it seems so strange. Of course, in the morning, if you have no experience with your dream symbols, you won't understand the meaning of this dream, and no dream dictionary will be able to provide you with the right interpretation! Your body will continue to inform you, with the same dream theme or with other themes or symbols like the following:

You dream of spitting out frogs, small snakes, and toads, like the witches of fairy tales.

You dream that you are at a banquet, you are very hungry, and all the other guests have been served except you, and the hunger becomes so unbearable that it sometimes wakes you up.

You often dream of groups of grayish people walking through corridors or labyrinths. In symbolic dreams, dark colors, and especially everything grayish, refer to all that has little energy compared to your own. Such is the case with intestinal parasites, which do not have a high level of life-energy compared to that of a normal healthy human. Thus, in our dreams, intestinal worms can appear as groups of gray figures or shadows walking in corridors that symbolically represent our intestines.

You often dream that you are ravenous and always in desperate search of something to eat. In addition, you may also be forever hungry in the waking state, and before falling asleep, you have the habit of dwelling on what you are going to eat the following day. (Normally, except, perhaps, in the case of chefs, we don't tend to think about food when we go to bed. Instead, we generally "digest" all the information and experiences of the day.)

These examples are not exhaustive. It is up to you to do personal work to find out how your body signals the presence of parasites in your digestive system. Thanks to this, you will learn to detect which of your common dreams are informing you of this predicament.

Thanks to scientific research, we now know that there is a link between the functioning of our "two brains," that is, the one in our head and the one in our belly. It has been scientifically proven that the state of the intestinal flora affects our mental health, and that intestinal dysbiosis can sometimes cause serious psychological issues. Intestinal flora transplants are now performed to help people recover their health. Of course, if I were a doctor and consulted by a person with a healthy lifestyle but some digestive or mental problems, I would first check for the presence of parasites in the digestive tract. But hey, why wait until we are so sick, when thanks to our dreams, we can detect the presence of parasites at the earliest stages of infestation and act quickly to avoid big damage?

If you have pets, you have certainly observed how their mood and vitality improve dramatically after a deworming. Indeed, it is common to see adult dogs, who have remained inactive for a long time, resuming playing after a successful deworming. This incredible improvement in mood and health also occurs in people who eliminate parasites from their bodies. There is no need to take my word for it, but you can find out for yourself.

Many people, including some doctors, are shocked and disgusted by the idea that they may host parasites, and they choose not to countenance the thought. Like it or not, take action, because long-lasting inaction in this case could cost you so much energy that you may sink into an inexplicable and deep depression!

Another cause of excessive energy expenditure stemming from nutrition is linked to stress.

c) Eating under stress or in negative emotional state is bad for your energy

When you are angry, wait until the anger is gone before you start eating because anger interferes with the proper functioning of the liver, preventing good digestion. Undigested foods create toxins in the body. Chinese acupuncturists have observed that an energetically disturbed liver triggers anger and, of course, disturbs digestion.

There are five sphincters along our digestive tract, and their functioning can be disturbed by stress and negative emotions. Knots in the stomach or fear in the belly prevent us from digesting well. Stress hinders the correct assimilation of food and temporarily slows down or blocks the correct elimination of waste. To get rid of this overload of waste, the body has to expend a lot of energy. The food intake that was deemed to restore the body energy in fact depletes it if we eat in an emotional state that disturbs digestion.

In waking life, we may be unaware of our permanent state of stress because we are used to our hectic routines. But our dreams never fail to sound the alarm bell to inform us about this high amount of stress disturbing the body. It is up to us to pay them more attention and take action to avoid stress-related health issues!

Here are some common themes of dreams about stress which show up long before the dreamer becomes aware of this stress in his waking life:

You dream of losing control of your car or any other vehicle.

You have some light nightmares, like losing your bag or your credit card.

You dream of having to take a train or a plane and facing a multitude of obstacles. For example, you have forgotten your suitcases, you no longer know where the airport is, you have forgotten your passport, etc.

Your dreams can use many other themes and symbols to show you that you are under too much stress. Each person is different, and it is up to you to undertake personal dream observation work to find out which of your dreams relate to stress. Detecting this kind of dream is vital because at this earlier stage it is much easier to recover your balance. A little rest, some relaxing herbal tea, a walk in the midst of nature, or deep breaths may be enough to help you quickly counteract the impending body or mind imbalance and avoid energy loss.

In summary, the very same nutrition which should always bring us energy can sometimes deplete it. If this occurs too often and for too long, it may lead to depressive states. The good news is that our dreams can help us avoid reaching this point because they always warn us as soon as our digestion and/or our elimination systems are not working properly. Poor elimination can also decrease the efficiency of the digestive system and lead to a buildup of toxins in the body. Now let's take a look at a second common activity that can drain our energy.

2) When and how does sexuality drain our energy?

We all know that to stay healthy it is best to avoid excesses. Sexual excess is no exception to this rule, and it is known that it can cause depletion of vital energy and thus be conducive to depression. What is less known is that, even without excess, under certain circumstances, sexual activity can deplete the vital energy of one, or both, of the partners and can lead to depressive states. We will see below why this is possible.

What happens when we have sex? What is it for?

Modern science answers these questions with reference to anatomical knowledge and some psychological considerations related to pleasure, emotions, and reproduction.

But if we commit ourselves to observe through our dreams what happens energetically in our body when we have sex, we will discover a new and different dimension of sexual activity that has not yet been explored by science.

Through observing our dreams and experimenting, we can observe that we are more than physical bodies: we are also immaterial beings, and we absorb, transform, and emit energy and information. We are surrounded by an energy field which also contains information. This energy field, called "aura" in some spiritual traditions, was photographed by the Russian researcher Semyon Kirlian.

Clairvoyants can perceive this aura that surrounds every human being, and we are all capable of seeing it in the dream state clearly or symbolically through the color of the characters' clothing.

From my personal research, I have come to the conclusion that when two people meet, an exchange of energy and information occurs between their energy fields; each person picks up some energy and information from the other. We actually constantly exchange information and energy with the people around us, whether we are aware of it or not.

During sex, this exchange is much deeper. In addition to the exchange of information and energy linked to the proximity of the bodies, there is a discharge of sexual energy during the orgasm. This sexual energy is also filled with a lot of information. I am not asking you to believe me implicitly but to do your own experiments and to make use of the dream state to observe better the changes that occur in your energy and information field as a result of sexual activity. You will be able to see in your dreams how much we charge ourselves with the energy and thoughts of our sexual partner, so much so that sometimes we can even dream of being in her/his body, and experiencing all her/his physical sensations.

Sex can be beneficial to both partners and can even recharge both of them if they reach orgasm at the same time, have similar energy levels, a compatible energy vibration, positive thoughts during sex, and, most of all, love for their partner. Furthermore, sexual intercourse must take place in an energetically healthy and favorable place.

Nowadays, these conditions are seldom met, and sexuality almost always depletes the energy of one of the partners, and sometimes of both.

In the waking life, if a person with a high level of energy meets a person with a lower level of energy, she will automatically transfer some of her energy to the person with a lower energy. Within a couple, this effect of communicating vessels between the "more alive" and the "less alive" is amplified by sexual intercourse. In other words, if a man and a woman live together and have sex regularly, over time they harmonize their energies and vibrations and form a new energetic entity. Everything is fine if in the beginning the energies of the two partners were equivalent in quantity and quality. Instead, if one partner was much more alive than the other, the harmonization is detrimental to him, and he may feel depressed if the couple's overall energy is below the usual energy level he had when single. This is a common state of affairs, and people who have become depressed after a "happy marriage" should check if they are losing too much energy in married life by getting away from their partner for a while.

If you are the person who is losing energy in the couple, and if this is the cause of your depression, you will learn so very quickly from your dreams as soon as you take some "vacations" from married life. In this case, the bright colors and dynamic themes will flood back to your dreams, and you will soon feel in a better mood in the waking state. People who love you but have a much lower energy level decrease your energy even if you love them in return. Unfortunately, some people who wish you the best with all their heart and soul can sometimes drain so much of your energy that you can fall into depressive states if you spend too much time with them, or, even worse, if you have sexual intercourse with them.

But depression is not, alas, the only consequence of a bad emotional association; sometimes it also happens that, immediately after marriage, disease strikes one of the partners and sometimes both.

Botanists know that some plants associate well with each other and work together, while others are incompatible with each other. The same is true for animals, and also for humans.

To avoid forming an energetically harmful couple, instead of relying on our usual criteria, we should choose a suitable partner from the point of view of vitality, that is, someone with an energy level equivalent to ours and a compatible vibration. If we can't find one, it is much better not to be in a relationship and to limit sexual intercourse as much as possible. If we have sex in these circumstances, some time spent alone will be necessary to compensate for the energy loss.

By observing your dreams, you will know who your partner is from an energetic point of view. You will also see how your energy varies with continuous contact with another person and especially when you have sex. Later on, I will speak about the changes occurring in our dreams whenever our energy starts to fall.

Obviously, we must take into account the entire life circumstances of couples; there may be other reasons that can lead one partner or the other to get depressed. These reasons may encompass changes in lifestyle, diet or home. And it is well known that some homes can severely disturb the energy of their inhabitants.

3) Energy losses caused by the home

While I was in Mexico, I saw all kinds of plants that don't grow in my country, and it made me think that like them, human beings thrive better in some places and feel bad in others. This aspect of life is essential. The place where we live, and especially the room where we sleep, has a tremendous influence on our physical and mental health.

We constantly exchange information and energy with others and also with our environment. Some places may be favorable, neutral, or harmful to our psychological health because, just like certain people, they may not be suitable for us through their disharmony with our energy fields and personal vibrations. Everyone perceives a certain environment in their own way and has a personal reaction to it.

Whenever I find myself in a place that has a vibration that disturbs me, I sense it immediately, and if I can, I hasten away from it. Thanks to all my work on dreams, I have greatly developed my sensitivity and perceptions in the waking state, to the point that I can quickly detect good and bad energy in homes and other places. You, too, can develop this ability—it is not difficult. In the meanwhile, here are some tips that will help you.

a) Clues to beneficial habitats perceivable in the waking state

When we are in a place that is beneficial to our energy field, we tend to be in a good mood, want to have fun, and feel good, creative, relaxed, and playful. In these places, artists, and writers are inspired and can focus easily on their work.

People with long hair can easily observe how they react to different environments. In a supportive environment, your hair grows faster and looks better; the same goes for the nails. In energetically unfavorable places, you may be stuck with bad hair all the time.

In places with good energy, we fall asleep quickly and wake up in a positive mood after a calm night of uninterrupted sleep. We dream easily and have pleasant dreams. We feel relaxed and refreshed after a good night and love spending time at home.

Some sensitive people are aware of the beneficial influence of their environment when they are awake.

Unfortunately, many people perceive nothing about the energy of their habitat when they are in the waking state. Their bodies automatically collect information about their environment and its energy, but this information cannot reach their conscious minds. Fortunately, such information can still seep into their minds through their dreams. An environment that is energetically harmful, even if we are unaware of it, is always a source of disturbance to the body, which never fails to signal this through dreams. People who do not consciously sense the harmfulness of certain places, and who do not pay attention to their dreams, remain in such bad environments instead of moving elsewhere. For a while, everything is fine, as they draw on their energy reserves, but gradually a state of tiredness and malaise sets in. Most of the time, people resort to consulting doctors, never suspecting for a moment that the cause of their problems may be linked to their home, especially when they find it very beautiful and attractive from an aesthetic point of view.

b) Clues perceptible in the waking state regarding harmful habitats

This is obviously the exact opposite of what happens in a beneficial habitat. In a habitat whose energy disturbs our body, we tend to be sad, depressed, and to feel lonely, isolated, and trapped. Artists have a hard time getting to work and finding inspiration. Children are loath to do their homework or have difficulties concentrating.

We have less determination in facing life, less enthusiasm for entrepreneurship, less desire to discover or learn. Sleep is less restful, and falling asleep is more difficult. Getting out of bed in the morning is a tragedy! When the energy is very disturbed, we can become sleepless or, if we manage to sleep, we can suffer from terrible nightmares. If we have long hair, it is easy to observe that in this environment it becomes flatter, dull, and brittle. In some living spaces, we may feel trapped and have only one desire: to get the hell out of there. But at the same time, we may lack the requisite energy to do so, as we fall into a lethargic state.

Sometimes, the house as a whole is not harmful but merely the place where we sleep. Some cases of chronic insomnia are simply due to poor position of the bed, and it is enough to change its position to restore restful sleep without drugs. On the Internet, mattress and bed sellers have published articles dedicated to the best way to orient your bed so as to promote sleep, and you will also often find feng shui advice on their websites. However, the best way is to experiment by changing the position of the bed and furniture, and to observe its effects on your body, mood, sleep, and even dreams.

If you are depressed and/or have trouble sleeping, before you go to a doctor and take pills for the rest of your life, first check out if the cause of your problems may be your home. Try sleeping elsewhere; if by doing so, you sleep much better and feel more at ease, go back to your usual place and orient the bed in a different way or try sleeping in another room. You may find a more favorable location. If you can't do it on your own, consult a geobiologist, who will help improve the energy of your home. A good geobiologist will find ways to improve this energy or will advise you on bed placement. So many depressions, and even deadly illnesses, could be avoided if only there were more awareness about the energetic quality of our homes and the other places where we spend a lot of time.

In some buildings, all the inhabitants and even their pets get sick. You will find striking examples of this phenomenon in *The Geobiology Guide* by Michel Moine and Jean-Louis Degaudenzi. I develop this theme in my book *Tricks to Sleep Better*, where you will find examples related to environments such as mountains and streams, or the seaside. Such places are considered health-friendly, but they can also cause insomnia and destroy your holidays if the bed is wrongly positioned with regard to the powerful flow of energy in natural settings! Let's now see what happens when we start sleeping in places that are energetically harmful.

c) This is what happens in dreams when you move to an energetically unsuitable location (and/or place the bed in the wrong position for your energy)

Your body tells you in your dreams that it is tired, that something is bothering it, and, by triggering nightmares, it may insist on pushing you to act and change this situation.

In these places, it is more difficult to relax and therefore fall asleep. We can fall asleep right away only when we are extremely exhausted, and sometimes after a few hours we wake up and cannot go back to sleep.

After some time, you simply tend to forget your dreams because you sleep less and less. Your sleep becomes lighter and you have less energy available to keep your memory functioning optimally and thus recall your dreams. Finally, you come to have so little vitality that you are unable to fight infections effectively, and you become increasingly sick and depressed. Unfortunately, in these cases your doctors "cure" you with the usual drugs, without ever solving the root problem in your home. It really is a great pity!

Those who for some reason are nevertheless able to sleep "normally" in energetically harmful places often dream of sleeping or of being worn out, with an irresistible desire to sleep. They tend to have nightmares, find it difficult to get out of bed in the morning, and feel tired even after a reasonably long sleep. Unfortunately, they may eventually die without ever suspecting the cause of all their suffering.

The ancient builders of cathedrals, pyramids, churches, temples, and other public and private buildings had a firm knowledge of cosmo-telluric energies. They didn't just build anywhere, willy-nilly. The shape of the buildings was not based purely on aesthetics; instead, it was chosen from an energy point of view. The ancient architects obeyed the natural laws of energy to erect buildings that were favorable to human life. Such natural laws seem to have ended up in oblivion, and our modern architects are forced to comply with bureaucracy and financial issues rather than the laws of nature, good health, and life. To this day, some ancient buildings have maintained such a high energy that it is no coincidence that so many tourists want to visit them. Even materialists and atheists are attracted to them and feel alive there. If you are depressed, pay a visit to some of these ancient buildings; they could help you heal. If you wish to delve deeper into this topic, I refer you to my book cited above. Let's now turn our attention to a third way of losing a lot of energy: the human environment.

4) Loss of energy caused by the people around us: energy vampirism

As I said, we all have both a physical and an energetic dimension, and the body is surrounded by a field of energy made up of all of our emanations. When we observe our dreams in a certain way, we become aware that we constantly receive, transform, and emit energy and information, and cognizant of the way this phenomenon varies according to different locations and the people we meet.

Previously, we talked about the energy losses which can occur when we have sex with someone who has a lower energy level than ours. This phenomenon of communicating vessels also occurs, but to a lesser extent, during non-sexual interactions.

When people meet, their energy fields meet too, and a flow of energy and information occurs between them. We commonly consciously perceive only a very small fraction of all the information collected by the body and the subconscious mind during an encounter with someone. But if you pay attention to your dreams, you will perceive in them information belonging to other people with whom you have been in contact. Dreams can also contain information from strangers, for example, from people who have traveled next to us on a train or a plane. Hence the difficulty of interpreting certain dreams made up of heterogeneous information, but that's another story!

Whenever someone drains your energy, your body and your subconscious mind inform you of the fact. This person may appear in your dreams as invasive plants, threatening animals, or as people you have known in the past that also drained your energy. In severe cases, the subconscious mind can provoke terrible nightmares to alert your conscious mind.

When intuition is not yet developed, there can sometimes be a surprisingly sharp contrast between how we evaluate a person with our conscious minds and with dreams and the subconscious. You should always trust the evaluation of your subconscious mind because it is never less than accurate, tells only the truth, and is not influenced by lies, social status, nice makeup, expensive clothing, or flattering appearance. The more you develop the communication between your conscious and subconscious minds, the harder it is to deceive you with lies and a dissemblingly beautiful appearance. You will be able to tell directly in the waking state what sort of a person you are dealing with.

When a person is experiencing negative emotional states, her energy is lower than usual. Therefore, even if this person does not want to bother others with her problems, she nevertheless influences their energy. Most of the time, we instinctually shrink from people who have an energy level which is too low for us, or who are experiencing energy disturbances due to negative emotions. So, whenever we are the one who is going through these negative states of mind, it is better to stay on our own and wait until we feel better to visit our friends.

As for people who are permanently deeply depressed and actively seeking the company of others for their own energetic advantage, we all instinctively want to distance ourselves from them immediately. If we fail to do so, we soon experience some physical and psychological signs of a drop in energy, even if the person is very kind, compliments us a lot, and claims she loves us.

Here are some of the more common physical signs of energy loss caused by someone draining your energy: you may suddenly feel hungry, want to have a snack, or indulge in one of your vices (cigarettes, alcohol, tea, or coffee, for example). You may feel a knot in your solar plexus, anxiety, or fear without reason. You may feel bored or lonely.

Once your depressed interlocutor is sufficiently recharged at your expense, she has only one idea: to be on her way. At that point, she abruptly ends the conversation with a good excuse to leave. Instead, you are left feeling a kind of void, and you instinctively feel the need to stay with her a little longer. But she scarpers even if you insist that she remains, because if she stays any longer with you, after a while the energy flow would be in your favor again. You would absorb back the energy that you gave her and that she would waste as usual.

This person will also come back to you as soon as she needs a recharge and will be so very happy and enthused to see you again provided that, in the meantime, you have recharged yourself correctly; otherwise, she will immediately look for energy elsewhere.

Depressed people who are unaware of their condition and have developed a habit of recharging from others from a young age often also have a tendency to waste their energy! They sense the energy level of others with remarkable efficiency and immediately turn to the best and most accessible sources of supply.

If, for some reason, you find yourself temporarily in a depressed state, this type of person instinctively keeps away from you, even if until the day before they have actively sought your company as one of their richest sources of supply. Even if you have helped them many times throughout their life, they run away from you whenever you are the one facing a problem for a change and in need of some help. It is not a question of morality or ingratitude; it is a purely instinctive attitude.

Today many human beings have an energy level which is so low it borders on depression without being aware of it. These people can be more harmful than those who are aware that their energy is too low and seek a cure for their problems instead of going to recharge themselves on the energy of others. Sometimes, they are difficult to detect while you are awake, but your dreams always tell you if you are associating with "vampires." And if you have too low an energy level, your dreams let you know, and show you how to right this situation.

We all must seek to get to know ourselves better and not behave like vampires when we are in an energy deficit.

50

Instead, we must make use of our dreams to avoid wasting our energies and learn how we can recharge ourselves better.

If there were an instrument capable of measuring human vitality, it would be appropriate to take this measurement after a period of isolation because our personal energy levels vary depending on whether we are alone or with other people. For example, if a person has a high level of energy because she usually benefits from that of a group of people (for example, a political leader, team leader, mother with many children, singer, or teacher), her level of energy will drop dramatically when she is isolated for a while and therefore relies only on her own reserves. Conversely, people who are usually drained by those around them will see their energy level rise again when they spend time alone. At the beginning of isolation, a person who usually recharges herself at the expense of a group of other people is fine for a while and then begins to feel depressed as soon as she has exhausted her stock of energy. Instead, a person in the opposite situation usually has difficulty being alone at first, but as soon as she has recharged herself adequately, she finds that she feels much better on her own and greatly appreciates this time of solitude.

This is pretty much how things work from an energetic point of view among human beings. It is up to you to record your own experiences and observations. Of course, sometimes other variables come into play. There are, for example, people who have such powerful energy that they can recharge others, even in large numbers, without any discomfort, through their ability to recharge themselves so quickly and abundantly. Often, they also are healers. Their healing may seem miraculous, but this is because we tend only to see the material side of existence. Instead, whatever is no longer functioning in the body due to a blockage in the flow of life-energy can immediately return to full function if that blockage is removed with an energy boost supplied to the system. This is not a miracle; it is just a simple natural law.

Even without speaking to you, a person can drain your energy with her mere physical proximity, but she can make it worse if she has negative thoughts about you.

Let's see now why thoughts affect the energy of living beings.

5) Loss of energy due to negative thoughts and the emotions they arouse

There is nothing easier than to experience the effects of thoughts and emotions on our physical health. Popular expressions such as "my guts are churning" and "I have a knot in my stomach" are very clear in this regard.

The French writer Honoré de Balzac was a sound observer of the phenomenon of thought and wrote the following:

"I wanted to reveal a secret to you; here it is: thought is more powerful than the body, it eats it, absorbs it and destroys it; thought is the most violent of all the agents of destruction, it is the true exterminating angel of humanity, which kills and vivifies, yes, it vivifies and kills. I have done my experiments several times to solve this problem, and I am convinced that the duration of life is due to the strength that the individual can put against thought; the fulcrum is the temperament. Thinking is adding flame to the fire."[2]

Before, all that was said about thoughts and their effects could only be subjective. Now, thanks to technological progress, it is possible to take an objective approach to the energetic reality of thoughts. For example, a few years ago, during a visit to an innovation fair, I saw in a booth an unexpected practical application of the power of thought. The inventors had had the brilliant idea of amplifying the waves emitted by the brain when we think so as to allow quadriplegics to be able to use a computer with the energy of their thoughts alone. This energy was picked up on the skull with electrodes and amplified.

Other researchers have investigated the effects of thought on water. Among them, Japanese researcher Masaru Emoto published several books with beautiful photographs showing how crystals of frozen water display more or less harmonious patterns according to the thoughts transmitted to the water. His laboratory and

---

[2] *Les Martyrs Ignorés,* Honoré de Balzac

specialist equipment allowed him to perform his experiments and take these pictures. Thanks to his books, we can all admire the beauty of water that has been influenced by positive thoughts, and we can be aware of the opposite effect of negative thinking. As water is so sensitive to our thoughts, it is no wonder that they have an incredible effect on our health, as our bodies are around 65% water.

Masaru Emoto's work was welcomed by mainstream media and many people heard about it. The French researcher Jacques Benveniste was not so lucky, and his life and career were ruined due to his work on the memory of water. I hope that one day the scientific community will do him justice, as well as so many other inventors and researchers whose discoveries were contrary to the scientific dogmatism of their time and/or certain financial interests. In France, research on the memory of water has been resumed by Professor Luc Montagnier, Nobel laureate, who has claimed that Jacques Benveniste was right about the memory of water.

You, too, can conduct interesting experiments on the properties of water informed by your thoughts and emotions. For example, you can hold a glass of water in your hands, then focus your mind on the point in the center of the forehead and direct your thoughts or images through this point to the water. Once you have informed the water in this way, you can drink it just before going to bed and mentally express the desire to perceive the effect of this water on your body in a dream.

Almost all spiritual traditions worldwide have taken into account the importance of right thinking and have implemented individual or group practices, such as praying or reciting mantras, so that individuals can use this faculty of their minds to enhance their vibrations.

Nowadays, we attribute less and less importance to the power and content of our thoughts, so much so that many are unaware of the disastrous effects that some books, movies, or songs have on their health. This is not to mention the effects of all the shocking news circulated by mainstream media every instant. Instead of indiscriminately accepting any manner of information to "feed" ourselves as if we were eating junk food, we should rather choose the intellectual and emotional foods that are most conducive to our health and that can help increase our energy. Do we not select our foods carefully and reject all that is inedible? If there is one thing I recommend above all others for depressed people, it is to avoid depressing books, movies, videos, and other content that is detrimental to their energy and their emotions. Depressed people are living in the middle of a toxic cloud of their negative thoughts that attracts more negativity to their lives and leads them to negative "intellectual foods," worsening their situation. Instead, they should look for anything that can help them break this vicious circle of negative thinking that in turn attracts further negative thoughts, people, problems, and events.

We should do positive thinking exercises every day in the morning after getting up and also before going to bed, and choose our intellectual foods wisely. These should increase our energy and improve our mood and well-being, instead of bringing in negative emotions like anger or sadness that drain energy, feed on themselves, and so initiate a vicious circle.

We have now seen the main and most frequent ways we can expend too much energy, namely, nutrition, sex, certain interactions with others, and thoughts and emotions. Of course, we also lose energy when we work or exercise. Everybody knows this, and we also know that working too much or doing too much exercise is harmful to our health and should be balanced with regular rest. Choosing the right activities is also of prime importance. Who hasn't experienced how much more energy is wasted doing a job we don't like or a sport we don't enjoy?

Now let's turn our thought to the best ways to gain energy.

CHAPTER 2: How We Can Gain Energy

1) Learn how to stop wasting energy on activities where energy is most frequently lost

First of all, you can gain energy, instead of losing it, by making wise choices about the everyday activities we have seen above: nutrition, sex, way of thinking, exchanges with others, home, work, and sport. Even if you have been leaking energy in these activities for a long time, it is never too late to change your habits and gradually reverse the situation to your favor.

I refer you to my book on dreams and health, which will help you make smarter choices with the help of your dreams.[3] You will also benefit greatly from websites that provide advice on natural nutrition, fasting practices, and alternative medicine. You will have no problem finding videos, websites, and books about these topics on the

---

[3] *Your Dreams Can Save Your Health*, Anna Mancini

Internet. You will also find that there are followers of all types of diets. To find out which diet is the most suited to you, you can experiment with the help of your dreams and close observation of your body. Eventually, you will discover which one is right for you. But remember, this can vary over time, depending on the season and place, so always listen to your dreams and your body to constantly adapt your diet.

2) Connect to the most powerful energy source

Some depressed people, who have not understood or do not want to understand how they could fix their depression, have acquired, more or less consciously, the habit of recharging themselves at the expense of other people. This is obviously energetic vampirism, a much more common phenomenon than we imagine. It frequently occurs within couples, and some people think they are in love with their partner when they only need her/his vitality, without which they would feel awful.

Yet there are ways to change, to become energetically self-reliant, and to have true loving relationships with others instead of just depending on their energy. The most powerful of these consists in restoring communication with the "inner self" by paying close attention each morning to our dreams. Dreams are the main channel through which we can liaise with the inner self. The simple fact of getting up quietly in the morning and starting the day by calmly writing down your dreams is a sort of meditation that brings out key emotions, memories, and sensations. This simple personal work not only helps restore communication between your inner self (your super consciousness, your soul, your higher self, or whatever you call it) and your conscious mind but also contributes to dissolving energy blocks and improving the circulation of life-energy within the body.

Thanks to this early morning personal work, you will gradually be able to remember your dreams more easily. After a period of practice, you will no longer want to start the day without this little ritual because its effects will be so life enhancing.

By observing your dreams and how they relate to your reality, you will come to know your body and mind better.

Dreams will show you if you have psychological issues and help you fix them. The fewer psychological blocks you have, the better the energy can circulate within your body, and this also contributes to improved communication between your conscious mind and your inner self. Rebuilding the broken bridge between your conscious mind and your higher self will allow you to open the door wide to your own source of energy, a personal spring which is abundant and inexhaustible. You will be able to tap into this powerful source when you are in the dream state, and you will wake up in the morning fully refreshed, inspired, happy, and with a wonderful zest for life.

Some creative activities carried out in the waking state, which vary from person to person, can also help reconnection to the inner self and help access this gushing spring of life-energy. The same is also true for meditation.

As you observe your dreams, you may notice that the conscious mind and its rationality tends to consume much more energy than it gives us. You will also find that when you act in accordance with the needs of your inner self, your dreams become more beautiful, colorful, and brighter, and you experience joy in your life, regardless of your material circumstances.

In other words, we can get the best energy recharge by acting in compliance with our deepest needs, those of our soul. But we need to know who we really are deep inside, what our real needs are, and what we have come to do in this world.

The answers to all of these questions pop up regularly in our dreams, but we usually pay no attention to them, especially when they don't seem to fit with our ambitions or with life choices we have made in the past.

The best way to have a high level of energy, which renders depression almost impossible, is to live a life in tune with our soul and its deepest needs.

At a certain point in my life, I received this advice in a dream: "Anna, do what you love and go where you are loved." This dream had been preceded by other recurring dreams which showed me that I was on the wrong path.

Staying on the "wrong path" is conducive to depression and other physical or mental health issues because, in the long term, the connection with the soul is lost, and therefore we can no longer rely on this potent spring of life-energy that is within us.

Here are some common themes of dreams which indicate to the dreamers that they are on the wrong path:

- Dreaming that we can no longer drive our car properly, or that we have great difficulty driving on a dark road where all is lost in the murk.

- Dreaming that our plane has crashed or that we have fallen from the top of a mountain, a hill, a high ladder, or a building can refer to the loss of spiritual ideals and the loss of contact with the inner self. This causes us to fall into a purely material life, with low vibrations, little spiritual life, and scarce energy.

- Dreaming of problems with bicycles, scooters, and other light means of transport frequently signals a loss of freedom due to poor life choices.

- Dreams of abandoned houses very often refer to what shamans call "soul loss." They invite the dreamer to rediscover his true path in life and reconnect to his deepest aspirations and to his soul.

Making life choices that fail to fulfill the needs and the purpose of the inner self is one of the things most conducive to depression. Avoid making life choices dictated only by financial, family, social, and other worldly considerations. Instead, to stay healthy, give priority to your deeper inner needs.

In the beginning, setting off down the wrong path may be experienced without discomfort. Unfortunately, this does not last, and after a while the person is gradually confronted by feelings of lack, of the void, and of being lost, and begins losing her zest for life, her enthusiasm, her brilliance, her inner beauty. She will become dull, less alive, less attractive to others, and most of the time all this will be attributed to aging.

For example, deep inside you are an artist, but through fear of poverty and failure, you decide to do a job that you despise because it brings you financial security. For some time, you may feel satisfied in spite of this choice. However, after a while, you will begin to notice some signs of energy deficit, such as boredom, loneliness, difficulty getting up in the morning, a feeling of emptiness, or even psychosomatic problems or chronic fatigue.

All this takes place because, little by little, you have cut the connection you had with your higher self as a creative person, and therefore you no longer benefit from its powerful supply of energy and its guidance. At some point, you may also start dreaming of abandoned houses.

Instead, in this converse example, if you have taken, despite the fear and obstacles at the outset, the path that your soul was dictating to you, you will almost always feel happiness, passion, pleasure in your work, and enthusiasm. All the activities that you perform with love will only serve to increase even further your energy and happiness instead of tiring you. You will be attractive, alive, true, and full of life until a ripe old age. It does not matter if on occasion you need a second job to support yourself: happiness is priceless!

Obviously, the ideal would be to live according to one's inner needs and, in so doing, also satisfy all the material needs of existence. But it takes so little, materially, when we do what we truly love. Happiness, good health, and longevity are the gifts of a life in harmony with the needs of our inner self. If material wealth could bring all that, there would be no suicides and depression among the world's richest.

Being mainly rational, our conscious mind is not well equipped to make the best choices. It can access only a limited amount of information, and it is far too influenced and programmed by our social environment. Instead, our inner self is much better equipped than our rational mind, and through our dreams it can guide us towards better life choices. As you get into the habit of observing your dreams, you will learn to tell very quickly if you have made bad life choices. Your dreams never fail to let you know if you are on a road towards decreased energy, depression, and other health issues. If you learn to understand your dreams, you will be able to take action immediately and avoid reaching a dreadful "dead end."

By warning us early of our "mistakes" and their consequences in terms of vitality, our dreams allow us to make better life choices and better manage our energy. For this purpose, dreams use a wide array of symbols, which vary from person to person. Everyone should do personal work to understand their personal dream symbols. However, regarding the onset of depressive states, there are some common warning signs, both in dreams and in reality, which apply to almost all of us. I will speak about them later.

If you are already depressed because you lost the connection with your higher self long ago, it is never too late, nor impossible, to regain your energy, but you may need an external energy boost to help you.

3) If you are already too depressed, seek outside help

When we are depressed, we vibrate at a frequency that attracts everything around us that vibrates at a similar frequency, that is, all depressing thoughts, people, and situations. This is a vicious circle that is sometimes extremely difficult to escape from without outside help.

Depressed people only see the negative side of all the solutions their relatives concoct to help them. They are particularly pessimistic and inactive. They no longer have the energy to shake off their condition on their own; sometimes they don't even have the strength to consult a doctor.

In this case, I advise family members and relatives to form a "help group" to support the depressed person with the energy of the group. It is best not to act alone, as there is a risk of becoming depressed instead of the person we wish to help. This is the principle of prayer groups, but you can also do it independently of any faith.

When I was in my twenties, as part of my research on human energy, I followed a healing group from northern France for several months. I went to their sessions as an observer, and then I did my survey of the people who had been treated there.

This group saw amazing results for all types of diseases, depression amongst them, but not in all patients. At the beginning of the session, the healers formed a circle holding hands and prayed that the sick would be healed. Subsequently, each healer laid hands on one of the sick people. Later on, I discovered through my research that it was not even necessary to be physically present and act on the physical body through the laying on of hands to benefit from the additional energy that is sent to us by a group of people willing to come to our aid. You can experience this for yourself by registering with one of the many prayer and healing groups that exist around the world. You can find them easily on the Internet, especially in the United States. In Europe and elsewhere, it is also the function of the church to say masses to help people in difficulty.

How to explain this phenomenon? I told you before that when two people meet, if one has much more energy than the other, after a while the energy of the more "alive" person is transmitted to the other as a result of the phenomenon of communicating vessels. Likewise, the energy of a group can be intentionally transmitted to a specific person. The advantage of a well-formed group is that it generates much more energy than the sum of the individual energies of each participant in the group.

It is not so difficult these days to form a group to help a depressed person remotely. To conclude on external help, I would like to emphasize how interesting acupuncture is in preventing or relieving depression. It allows the energy to circulate better in the body, unblocks the existing "knots," increases vitality, and greatly improves mood. In addition, by transferring a little of his own energy to the patient, the acupuncturist helps balance her energy. Nature and especially trees can also help you with their life-energy. When you feel depressed, walks in nature, deep breaths, and sunbathing will do you a lot of good. Flowing water also has a relaxing and recharging effect on our bodies. When we bathe in the sea, especially at the end of the day, we benefit from all the solar energy that has been accumulated in the water throughout the hours of sunlight.

Obviously, you should not rely all the time on other people for a boost to feel better. It should be a one-off to give you the little extra energy you need to thrive on your own on your path to recovery. Otherwise, you will become a burden to others and never learn how to solve your problems. Once you have benefited from external help to boost your energy, the first thing you should do is to clean up your mind and, above all, change all the sources of information habitually harming your energy.

4) Change your sources of information

I spoke earlier about the effect on the human body of thought and emotions. Almost all current mainstream media is continuously spreading depressing and frightening information together with shocking images. The pandemic has further accentuated this trend. In France, it has had a catastrophic effect on mental health, and Eric Caumes, head of the infectious diseases department at the Pitié-Salpêtrière Hospital in Paris, told BFMTV on November 15, 2020: "The rate of depression is soaring among the general population, from 10% in late September to 21% in early November. It doubled in six weeks."[4]

He claimed that this increase was caused by the restrictions related to confinement. Lockdowns and all the limitations of freedom imposed during the COVID pandemic were certainly conducive to depressive states and nervous breakdowns for many people. However, some people used these apparently adverse conditions to increase their energy. I am one of them and during the lockdowns I relaxed, wrote new books, thought about my life, and took care of my body. But in order to feel good throughout that time, I cut myself off from all the frightening news that mainstream media was constantly disseminating. Under normal circumstances, I tend to scan the news briefly on the Internet. But this time, I soon

---

[4] https://www.rtl.fr/actu/debats-societe/coronavirus-un-infectiologue-alerte-sur-une-forte-hausse-du-taux-de-depression-7800923174

realized that I had to stop reading the news completely and instead focus my mind on positive thoughts to escape the "toxic cloud" created by mainstream media and the fear it aroused in populations worldwide. It is no surprise that the rate of depression has increased dramatically during the pandemic, and this is mainly due to the incredible morass of toxic fear created by so many people under the omnipresent influence of terrifying news from mainstream media and governments.

In the past, before the internet existed, I used to avoid putting up with the negative energies of the media by asking my family and friends to pass on only important and essential information, and also positive and uplifting news. Positive information is almost inexistent in the mainstream media; as for general news, there is little essential information, and most of it is false, distorted, and stressful. I got more accurate information by reading the parliamentary debates and the texts of the laws enacted on the subjects I was interested in.

The media industry is increasingly aimed at propaganda and spreading fear and negative emotions. They undermine the morale of entire populations to the point that I sometimes wonder whether their purpose is to help big pharma sell more anti-depressants.

So, if you are depressed, you should better protect yourself from this crippling effect of mainstream media and be smart in organizing yourself to get the news you need without having to cope with stressful, inessential news and the emotionally shocking images that accompany it. It is easy now to use some Internet-based services to sift out the information that interests you and discard all the rest.

Do not watch or read the news while you eat or immediately after meals. Even if you don't believe it to stress you out, with a little self-observation you will notice that it has an insidious effect deep inside you, and that it actually disturbs your digestion, affects your mood and your thoughts, and lowers your energy.

Today's most popular media have completely moved away from their informative role and have become tools of propaganda, disinformation, and manipulation. As long as this goes on, the best we can do from an individual and collective point of view is to ignore them and turn to other more objective, respectful, truthful, and positive sources of information. Moreover, once you are a trained dreamer, you can get all the important and true information you need directly from your soul and in your dreams.

Our bodies and our minds need truth. Lying is no good to anyone from an energetic point of view. The ancient Egyptians long ago observed that lying brings disease and poverty to individuals and societies. This is something you can easily verify by observing how much your muscle tone decreases when you lie.

Now let's take a look at some early signs of energy loss.

CHAPTER 3: Easily detectable early signs of energy drop

Before I talk to you about the most common dream signs of loss of vitality, I would like to start with a brief reminder of what normal sleeping and dreaming should be like for healthy human beings.

1) What constitutes normal sleeping, dreaming, and awakening?

<u>a) The normality of sleeping</u>

Normally, you should sleep deeply throughout the night, without having to get up several times to go to the bathroom. If you need to do so, there is a problem in your body that needs to be addressed, unless, of course, if you have drunk a lot of fluids before going to bed. At the beginning, this problem is often simply caused by congested and gas-filled intestines compressing the bladder. When the intestines are in such a state, they take up too much space in the belly to the detriment of all other

---

77

organs, including the bladder. Gas can also result from poor digestion or from having a heavy meal just before going to sleep.

b) Normality regarding dreaming

You should be able to remember your dreams easily, especially those you had on the point of waking up. Your dreams should be vivid, colorful, and bright. They should help you solve the current problems in your daily life and inform you about the state of your body. They should also project you into your future: that is, in the dream state, you should, under normal conditions and almost every night, see a little bit of the near future. Let's look at these different points in more detail.

Dreams should project you into your future

I have observed that one of the most important functions of dreams is to "build" our future. I am not the only researcher to notice this interesting function of dreams; Edgar Cayce also observed it, going on to conclude that everything we experience in our waking life was first conceived in our dreams.

By observing your dreams and their connections with your reality, you too can verify that, contrary to what is commonly admitted, it is not the conscious mind at the helm of our existence but our higher self. Sure, the conscious mind plays an important role in our waking life, but it is the higher self that subconsciously builds our reality, sometimes far in advance and with quite startling accuracy.

I have observed that each night my dreams shape my future for the next day. I have also noticed that some events I have lived showed up in my dreams clearly and accurately long before they actually occurred. Some events were "programmed" in my dreams ten years before they happened in my waking life; for example, my higher self had planned my stay in New York and what I would do there ten years earlier.

A small portion of your dreams should show you your psychological problems

In addition to creating our future, dreams also help us solve our problems of the past, psychological problems in particular. Normally you should have some psychological dreams here and there among the other dreams, especially during periods of rest and solitude. In fact, psychological dreams tend to be more frequent when we are not very active in waking life because our higher selves use the extra energy made available by inactivity, relaxation, and rest to "repair" our lives, our psyches, and even our bodies.

The more psychological problems you solve, the more energy you will have for other types of dreams, hence the importance of doing inner work to know yourself and to get rid of your old psychological blocks. By observing your dreams, you will be able to become fully aware of your emotional blocks and wounds and your psychological traumas, sometimes buried deep inside and sapping your energy. You will be able to release the energy that was feeding these blocks and benefit from it to increase your vitality.

Some dreams should regularly inform you about the condition of your body

When we are awake, the brain is constantly receiving information from all the parts of the body and from our environment. We are aware of some of the information sent by the body when it relates to unpleasant states such as pain, numbness, and chills. But a large quantity of information sent by the body to the brain does not reach our consciousness when we are awake. At night, this information can better reach our consciousness through our dreams. During sleep, the body sends information to the brain about its condition, good or bad, information which is conducive to forming symbolic or crystal-clear dreams. Such dreams are common and should occur regularly even when we are in good health. Generally, this is exactly what happens, but most of the time people are unaware of it through lack of understanding of their dream symbols. So, let's here mention briefly the most frequent symbols that can represent the body and its condition in our dreams: homes, nature, and cities. You will find detailed examples of such dreams and important information on how your dreams can help you better manage your physical health in my book: *Your Dreams Can Save Your Health, Signs of Infectious Diseases in Dreams, Dreaming the Right Remedies, Accurate Diagnosis, and Early Detection of Diseases.*

The different rooms of homes and the problems that appear there can represent symbolically the different organs of the body; for example, the kitchen corresponds to the digestive tract, the bathroom to the kidneys, the electrical system to the nervous system, the pipes to the veins, the attic and the roof to the head, the walls to the intestinal walls, etc. Nature, vegetation, rivers and the like can also stand in symbolically for the inside of the body. Finally, some cities we visit in the dream state and their condition, especially the state of the roads, also frequently represent the inside of the body.

<u>c) Normality regarding awakening</u>

When we are healthy, we wake up feeling refreshed and in a good mood. We don't need to motivate ourselves to get out of bed and go about our daily tasks. We effortlessly remember our dreams, especially those we have had just before waking.

Sometimes our dreams are interesting and help us start our day full of joy, new ideas, and beautiful visions. Such pleasant awakening is an indication of a good recharge and increased vitality in the body.

2) Early signs of energy loss and imbalances

We already have energy problems and are no longer normally healthy when we have:

- Troubled sleep, insomnia, or nightmares

- Frequent awakenings or overly light sleep

- Lack of or excessive sleep

- Difficulty falling asleep and getting up

- An almost total absence, for a long period of time, of dream memories

- Tiredness upon awaking and the need to take stimulants (tea, coffee...) to help start the day

- A persistent feeling of sadness and loneliness

- A feeling of boredom and emptiness towards life

- A feeling of lack of love. Often, people who are single believe that they have this feeling because they don't have a partner. Most of the time, they are off the mark, since this feeling is triggered by lack of energy in the body and can equally be experienced by married people. When we have a lot of energy, it is impossible to feel alone, or sad, or bored. This explains why some hermits can live alone for so many years in a state of bliss.

3) Early signs of decreasing energy in dreams

Whenever your energy starts decreasing, your dreams start changing. They gradually become less colorful, more repetitive, and less interesting. From a certain point, if we do nothing to remedy our energy decrease, dreams become increasingly dull, sad, and grayish.

There exists an important law regarding energy: the law of resonance. According to this law, we attract (in the world of dreams and also in the real world) everything that resonates with our level of energy, be it experiences, ideas, people, or situations. If our energy is too low, we attract unpleasant experiences, situations, ideas, sensations, and messages, and we are increasingly prone to stressful and unpleasant dreams and even nightmares. A vicious circle is established which sends us spiraling lower and lower.

People who are healthy should pay attention to their dreams so that they can take action as soon as their dreams show some early signs of decreasing vitality.

We should all make a good habit of observing our dreams regularly; it is the best investment we can make for our physical and psychological well-being. Thanks to dreams, we can learn to better manage our energy and to always keep it at a sufficient level to avoid depression and other health issues. Why become a prisoner of antidepressant drugs and their side effects and face such an ordeal when dreams are always there to help you as soon as something goes wrong inside?

I am a "trained dreamer," and should I be unable, for several days, to recall with ease a single dream, I immediately take action to remedy this situation. Of course, I am not at all willing to reach depressive states, nor am I interested in living without dreams. Without them, it would be like missing the most important half of my life. I have observed that this difficulty in remembering my dreams often stems from fatigue and poor diet associated with stress, and all I need to do is correct this as soon as possible. After that, my dream activity returns to normal.

With the exception of sudden severe traumatic events, we do not fall into depression overnight. Fortunately, our vitality declines gradually and not all of a sudden, and therefore depression needs some time to appear. For this reason, our dreams can help us avoid becoming desperately depressed because they allow us to take action to stem any loss of energy as soon as we observe it in our dreams. Of course, it is much easier to stop an incipient than an entrenched depression because, in the latter case, we no longer have enough energy and willpower to remedy the problem without external help.

There are so many well-known ways to help us restore our energy when we start losing too much of it. They range from resting, to better diet, fasting, walking in natural settings, sun and air bathing, sea water or thermal water baths, acupuncture, positive thinking, yoga, deep breathing, massages, and vitamins, amongst others. But there are also some little-known but efficient means to help increase our energy which were successfully used in France and elsewhere at the beginning of the twentieth century, when big pharma companies were not yet that powerful. Let's take a look.

CHAPTER 4: Some little-known technologies that can contribute to energy recharge and better health

1) The invention of the "Violet Ray" and its medical use

You have certainly heard of Nikola Tesla, famous throughout the world for his technological inventions.[5]

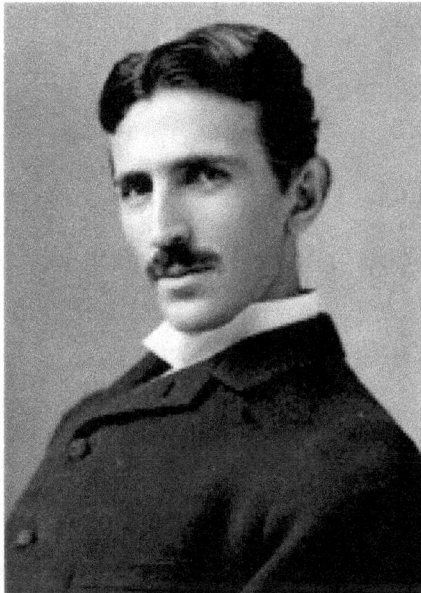

---

[5] Picture of Nikola Tesla
https://commons.wikimedia.org/wiki/File:Tesla_circa_1890.jpe

They changed the course of history to such an extent that most of our modern technologies are based on his discoveries. But you probably haven't heard of Tesla's medical inventions. One of them, the "violet ray", was popular in the United States among both doctors and the general public.

Around 1920 the violet ray was used by doctors to treat a wide variety of health conditions by stimulating life processes inside cells. The cells were stimulated by the high frequencies emitted by the violet ray, and the skin was disinfected by the ozone it produced, which is a natural disinfectant. The violet ray acts directly on the circulation of energy in the cells and therefore throughout the whole body.

https://youtu.be/iafoQ4b5cjo

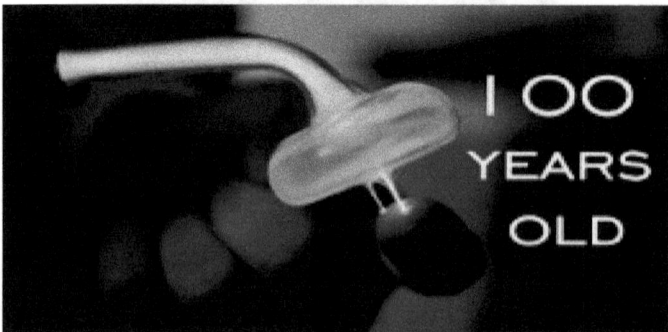

At the beginning of the twentieth century, the violet ray was sold throughout the United States. It was very affordable and was also available via the major mail order companies. The device used by doctors was a bit more expensive and sophisticated than the one sold to the general public. It came in a case with an assortment of electrodes of different shapes, intended for different internal and external parts of the body. You can see some pictures of them on the electrotherapy museum website:

http://electrotherapymuseum.com/MuseumVioletRay s.htm

The reports by doctors of the time on the successes they achieved, and on the treatment protocols they used, are very interesting and useful. I enjoyed reading some of them that I found on the Internet. In one of these reports, a doctor records his observation that after six months of daily use of the violet ray on the head of a patient, hair had regrown and recovered its natural color. [6]

---

[6] Eberhart, N.M. (1920). *A Working Manual of High Frequency Currents,* Chicago, IL: New Medicine Publishing Co., pp. 319

Unfortunately, after the war, some powerful pharmaceutical companies launched a propaganda campaign against the violet ray to dissuade the general public from buying this effective and inexpensive technology and prohibit its use by doctors.

Gradually, under the pretext of protecting people from the dangers of the violet ray, its manufacturers were taken to court, and producing violet rays was forbidden in the United States.

The media, in the pay of big pharmaceutical companies, had effectively spread their frightening lies and the idea that violet rays and ozone were harmful to health. They claimed that the violet ray caused severe damage, yet so many Americans had used it successfully for years! I previously mentioned a certain Edgar Cayce. In the hypnotic trance state, he could diagnose the origins of diseases with great precision and just as precisely prescribe the appropriate remedies. In more than 900 sessions, he recommended using the violet ray for the treatment of a wide variety of health issues. The reports of these sessions are still accessible and can be found at the organization he founded:

www.edgarcayce.org

Thanks to Cayce, knowledge about the beneficial health effects of Tesla's violet ray continued to circulate in the United States. Unfortunately, its manufacturing remained prohibited, and people had to import it from other countries.

Being of Serbian origin, Tesla regularly travelled to the countries of Eastern Europe, where he also spread knowledge of his inventions and the violet ray. While in the United States this fascinating device had gradually disappeared from circulation to be replaced by pharmaceutical drugs, it continued to be produced and used in most Eastern European countries. Thanks to them, the technological knowledge necessary to manufacture Tesla's violet ray became available all over the world.

Today, the violet ray is manufactured mostly in China and can be found in the cosmetics section of most major online shopping sites.

On YouTube there are many testimonials on the benefits of the violet ray on skin and hair, and, as far as I can tell, they are not censored because they do not present the violet ray as a medical device and brag about its health benefits. So, if you want to find information on how the violet ray can improve your physical and mental health, you must turn to the books that were published at the beginning of the twentieth century and the transcriptions of Cayce's sessions.

According to Cayce, the violet ray improves blood and lymphatic circulation where it is applied, and the ozone generated disinfects. (Ozone is increasingly used today to disinfect swimming pools, and in China, during the COVID epidemic, robots spraying ozone were deployed in Wuhan hospitals.)

I first heard about Tesla's violet ray thanks to Cayce. I hardly believed such results could be possible, but I decided to have a try with a cheap device, and I tested it on my skin and head. I can tell you without hesitation that the results are remarkable, both cosmetically and energetically.

Upon witnessing my own experiment and its excellent results, some friends adopted it too, and they also gave me positive feedback. I came to the conclusion that the violet ray demonstrates clearly that the health of human beings depends also on the good circulation of energy in their bodies, which in turn improves the flow of blood, nervous impulses, and lymph. The condition of the skin is visibly improved by the energy of the violet ray, and when I used it on my head, my mood immediately improved and my brain became more "active" to the point that I had to stop using it in the evening.

It is claimed that ideas are floating in the air just waiting to be plucked, and so it is common that patent applications for the same discovery are filed almost simultaneously by people in different countries. This frequent phenomenon occurred even when international communication was not so easy and did so with regard to the invention of the violet ray. While Tesla was busy inventing his violet ray in the United States, the Frenchman Jacques-Arsène D'Arsonval made the same discovery in Paris. You will find an interesting and detailed article about D'Arsonval on Wikipedia.[7]

In Europe, if you want to get your hands on this machine, now more commonly known as a "cosmetic device," it is easier to find it by searching on the Internet for "D'Arsonval" instead of "violet ray."

Tesla and D'Arsonval both demonstrated the importance of the energetic dimension of human health. They opened up a huge and promising field of scientific research into human energy and the healing use of energy. Following in their footsteps, many researchers have continued down this avenue of research. One of these was Georges Lakhovsky, who invented an interesting and highly effective machine. I have chosen to focus on Lakhovsky's

---

[7] https://fr.m.wikipedia.org/wiki/Arsène_d%27Arsonval

work because I find it so promising and intriguing, but if you want to know more about other enthralling inventions of the time, you can read the Wikipedia article on electrotherapy:

https://fr.m.wikipedia.org/wiki/Électrothérapie

2) Georges Lakhovsky's invention of the multiple wave oscillator and its successful use in French and Italian hospitals

Georges Lakhovsky was a Franco-Russian engineer who, in the 1940s, developed a multiple wave oscillator intended to restore health by energetically rebalancing the body cells. He was so successful in this endeavor that his oscillator was adopted by various French and Italian hospitals. Several doctors published reports on the cures they had obtained using the multiple wave oscillator on terminally ill patients.

You can read some of these medical testimonials in the books published by Lakhovsky himself.[8] You will also

---

[8] https://data.bnf.fr/fr/12617789/georges_lakhovsky/;
http://www.centrolakhovsky.com/it/libri.html

---

find them in many Italian medical publications of the time, which report many cases of apparently terminal cancers being cured. All this happened in the 1930s; in 1945 Lakhovsky fled from Nazi-occupied France and went into exile in the United States, where he continued his work. He died there in an accident at the age of seventy-five. Some believe this was, in fact, no accident but that he was killed because his inventions, like those of Tesla and other lesser-known inventors, were contrary to certain financial interests. Lakhovsky had been granted a patent for his oscillator, but after World War II, like Nikola Tesla's violet ray, his medical invention fell into oblivion.

To obtain a patent for an invention, an application must be filed with a patent office. Such a request must describe precisely the invention, how to realize it, and include expository technical drawings. Unfortunately, the patent filed by Lakhovsky was not detailed enough to allow the manufacture of his oscillator, and for a long time this valuable invention was considered permanently lost.

Fortunately, some oscillators in good working condition were found later on in Italy and the United States, and thanks to the reverse engineering they allowed, it was possible to start producing them again.

These machines are more complex, harder to use, and more expensive than Tesla's violet ray. Places where it is possible to have sessions with an oscillator are hard to find. In France, I have found only one, in a town near Paris.[9]

YouTube video showing Georges Lakhovsky's machine: https://youtu.be/QPX_dPCjk2U?

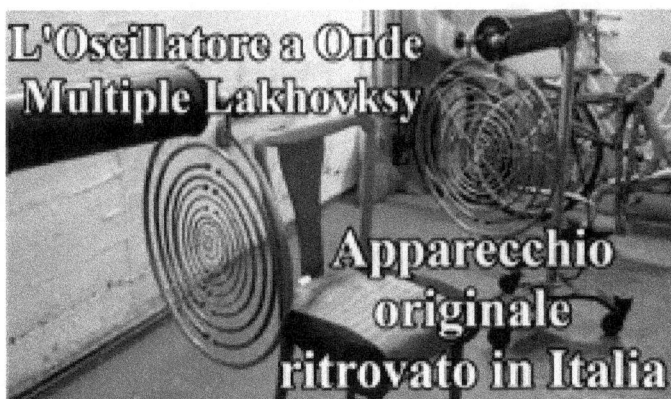

___

[9] Lakhowski's machine is available in Autun, France at «La boutique d'Agnès», http://www.bien-etre-boutique.com/boutique/

___

These oscillators also emit purple light; indeed, there are in line with the inventions of Tesla and D'Arsonval. In his book entitled *The Secret of Life*, Lakhovsky explains how the violet ray works and why it and the ozone it produces can cure many diseases. According to Lakhovsky, our cells vibrate at a certain electromagnetic frequency. When this frequency is disturbed, all kinds of pathologies are triggered. Lakhovsky proved that the places where we live can disrupt the functioning of the cells by disturbing their natural electromagnetic vibrations. He studied the correlation between the frequency of cancer onset and the nature of the soil and subsoil where patients usually lived, determining which types of soils and subsoils were favorable or harmful to health. I strongly advise you to read his books; they are very interesting and open up wider horizons on health and healing. Thanks to Lakhovsky's oscillators, people whose illnesses had been brought on by living in harmful places were able to restore their energy balance and recover their good health. The oscillator obviously made it possible to treat not only tumors and other serious diseases, but also depressions caused by energy loss due to electromagnetic disturbances in homes and other places the sick people frequented.

Lakovsky observed that human health is affected by cosmic vibrations, and that these vibrations are stored or reflected depending on the nature of the soil and subsoil and can cause energy disturbances in the human body. (For further reading, see his book Contribution to the Etiology of Cancer.)

It is clear to me that Georges Lakovsky and Nikola Tesla had rediscovered part of some ancient knowledge, and that their subsequent inventions resonate with ancient spiritual philosophies about the human being. Now I would like to talk to you about another means that you can use to increase your energy and avoid depression: water.

3) Vitalized water recharges the body's energy

Water plays an important role among all spiritual traditions, and many places of worship or pilgrimage have their "miraculous" springs. Whenever scientists have analyzed these miraculous waters, they have found that they do not differ from common waters. In my opinion, scientist have so far proved unable to detect a difference because they do not have the tools to measure the energy of water. Water from miraculous springs must be highly charged with cosmo-telluric energies, while common water is generally not. Whenever we drink water, we also drink the energy it contains. This energy can be favorable, neutral, or harmful to our energy system; in other words, the water we drink can recharge us with energy, drain us or, have no effect on us at all.

By using my dream faculties, and also observing the reactions of my body, I have experienced the effects of various thermal waters and other waters from different sites of Marian apparitions. Some thermal waters have done me a lot of good, and others have completely disturbed me. I have observed that some Marian waters increased my energy but not all of them. Whenever they did so, I became aware of it through the wonderful dreams they triggered—I was running full of strength and joy through stone buildings emanating magnificent energy, and in the morning, I felt renewed, fit, joyful, and recharged. I have also observed that some thermal waters have the same beneficial effect. If you are interested in the topic of Marian waters, you can read the works of Dr. Enza Ciccolo, who has conducted extensive research on them and invented protocols to use them effectively.

You will find interesting information and a link to her books on this site: **https://www.alaro.it/le-acque-a-luce-bianca/**

I have also experimented with the effect of solar water on plants and myself. I obtain such water by placing a transparent glass bottle of water in the sun with a tip of clear quartz at its top, the end in contact with the water. I have observed that this simple procedure significantly improves the taste of water and makes it more beneficial both for plants and for me. When I drink it before going to bed, it triggers the same types of dreams that I have obtained with Marian waters and with some thermal waters.

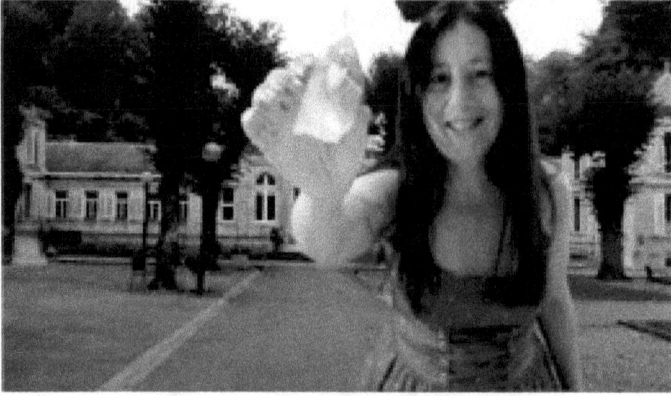

https://www.YouTube.com/c/LaSignificationdesRevesAutrement

I have posted a video on YouTube about the properties of quartz and some experiments I have done.[10]

You can also carry out experiments of your own. As you have seen, to test the properties of different waters, I have used the means available to me, that is, my body, my dreams, and plants. Instead, Marcel Violet, a French engineer, used technological means and invented a device to energetically charge water. He tested his vitalized water on a large scale on cultivated fields and entire herds of farm animals. His water allowed for more abundant

_____

[10] https://youtu.be/0eygq6waxRw

crops of fruit and vegetables, and kept farm animals much healthier.

You can find detailed reports of his experiences in his books.[11] Violet died in 1973, also as the result of an accident, but today you can still hear him talking about his experiences thanks to a YouTube video of a lecture (in French) recorded in 1962.[12]

https://www.youtube.com/watch?v=F_cNGAEElhA

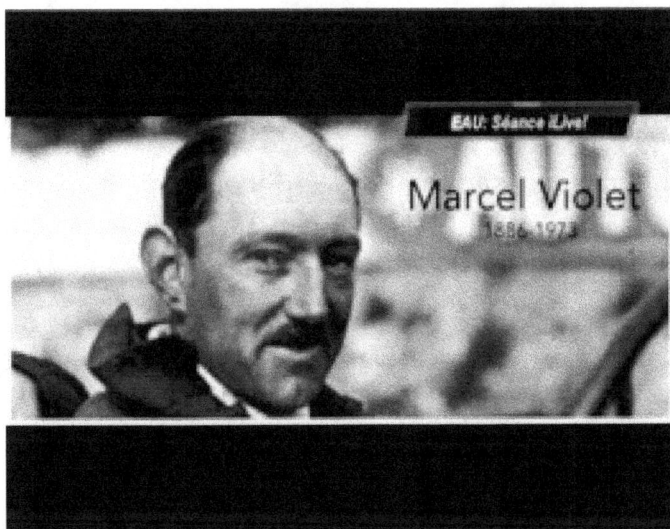

---

[11] Le Secret des Patriarches - Essai sur la Nature de l'Énergie Biologique
[12] Video Marcel Violet: https://youtu.be/F_cNGAEElhA

Violet created a company to manufacture and sell his device. Today it is still marketed, but by other companies. There have been many other devices to improve water invented; I find it captivating to read about the work of all these researchers, but sadly, their inventions and Violet's device are too expensive for most people.

If the topic interests you, you can read the works of Louis-Claude Vincent and Dr. Jeanne Rousseau on the website: **www.votre-sante-naturelle.fr**

You will find on YouTube some interesting interviews with Dr. Rousseau. She has invented bathtubs equipped with a device that creates whirlpools and vitalizes the water.

https://www.youtube.com/watch?v=Vl3aw5pM2pU

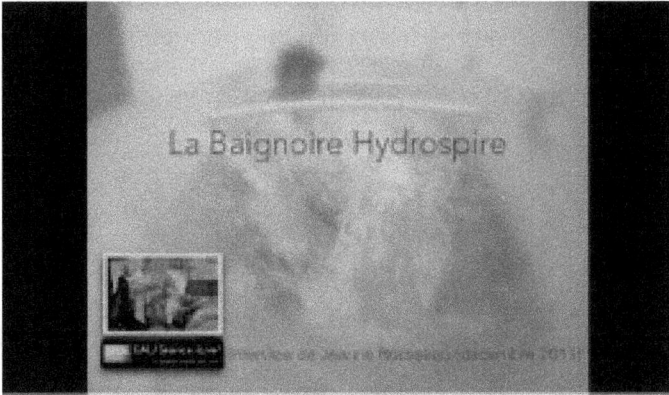

Water can also be charged with energy in the midst of nature and without any technology required. Indeed, when it flows through environments that are beneficial to our health, it picks up and stores these energies and we can benefit from such energy through drinking this water. This phenomenon may account for the healing effect of thermal waters and Marian waters, such as that of Lourdes.

For now, our bodies and dreams are still our best tools to understand whether we have gained or lost energy. I encourage you to develop your skills in the art of dreaming. Everybody can become a powerful dreamer, whatever their starting point. I have written many books to help you in this endeavor: simply choose the one aimed at your present level and then deepen your knowledge with others as you progress. Here there are:

For those who do not sleep well: Tricks to Sleep Better

For those who do not remember their dreams: *Tricks to Remember Your Dreams*

For those who dream but do not understand their dreams: *The Meaning of Dreams*

For those who wish to use their dreams to foresee their future: *The Clairvoyance of Dreams*

For those who wish to use their dreams in the field of innovation: *Scientific Creativity*

For those who wish to use their dreams in the archaeological field: *How to Unlock the Secrets, Enigmas and Mysteries of Ancient Egypt and Other Old Civilizations*

For those who wish to learn how to better manage their health through dreams: *Your Dreams Can Save Your Health: Signs of Infectious Diseases in Dreams, Dreaming the Right Remedies, Accurate Diagnosis, and Early Detection of Diseases*

For those who would like to understand what depression is, and how dreams can signal it when there is still time to avoid it: *Depression and How your Dreams Can Help You Avoid It*

You will find more information on my website: www.amancini.com

All of these books can be bought in online bookstores, in print, or as e-books.

CONCLUSION

Your dreams can help you understand better why and how you lose or gain energy, and such knowledge is a prerequisite to avoid or overcome depression. Fortunately, there are alternatives to anti-depressant medications and their terrible side effects. Paying close attention to your dreams can help you detect your "energy leaks" and their root causes at the earliest stage. They may stem from your diet, a clogged and parasite-infested digestive tract, an unhealthy sex life, disturbing energy in your home, energy-sucking people, and other factors. Depression can never be healed with pharmaceutical drugs that address the symptoms only; instead, it can be achieved when we find and fix the root cause that triggers our depressive states.

Negative thinking is an important cause of energy loss. Our thoughts and emotions can increase or decrease our energy. Edgar Cayce repeated often in his consultations that one must have "right thinking," to maintain good health. Living in hatred, anger, resentment, wickedness, or sadness means condemning ourselves sooner or later to becoming sick, because all these emotions weaken our energy and disturb our organs.

Dr. Edward Bach researched the links between negative emotions and pathologies thoroughly, and invented flower-based homeopathic remedies to help restore emotional and physical balance. Today, his remedies, known as "Bach Flowers," are easy to find in pharmacies and health food stores. However, many scientists make fun of people who believe in the effectiveness of these remedies, as is the case with homeopathy. Are they right?

The best way to find out the truth is to experiment with these floral remedies, and you can do so efficiently by using your dreams and observing your body. The subconscious mind and the body always tell the truth, and they need truth to flourish. The ancient Egyptians observed that lying is detrimental to the good health of people and countries because it slows down the flow of life and, in so doing, brings poverty and disease. They claimed that the gods hated lying above all. But lying, in ancient Egypt, also meant lying to oneself by not listening to the heart, that is to say, one's soul, higher self, and deepest needs. Through my research on the functioning of the human being at the junction of dreams and reality, I can say without a moment's hesitation that the ancient Egyptians were absolutely right.

And I would like to add a few words about Dr. William Bates, a New York ophthalmologist, who was unfamiliar with this ancient Egyptian thinking but observed through a retinoscope that uttering any lie immediately causes temporary loss of vision, even if the person does not know what she is saying to be untrue.[13]

It is so interesting to know our energy drops whenever we lie, even if we are unaware of not telling the truth. But where do we find the truth within us? The rational mind is highly prone to lying because it is too easily manipulated by all kinds of lies, propaganda, and beliefs. Instead, as the body and the higher self always tell the truth, and never make mistakes, they are our best friends

---

[13] *Better Eyesight Without Glasses*, William Horatio Bates

113

113

and guides throughout our lives. Most of the time, the rational mind is focused only on its own interests and is constantly making its little selfish plans. With our conscious minds, we tend to imagine that we can get away with anything in our behavior and in our relationships with others, but self-observation, especially through the dreaming process, shows very soon that we pay with our energy for all the bad uses we make of our conscious minds.

The conscious mind should always be at the service of the higher self to help fulfill our deepest and truest needs. When the conscious mind is no longer at the service of the soul, the doors of our powerful inner springs of life slam shut. It is up to us to choose how we want to live and what we want to prioritize, and then take the consequences in terms of quality of inner life, health, and well-being.

Let's end on an optimistic note. The ancient Egyptians, who were unfamiliar with the concepts of sin and guilt, claimed that it was always possible to correct our mistakes and restore the correct flow of Maat, that is, of vitality, in the body and in society. So, let's use all the means available to us to recover our energies and, above all, let's better understand the natural laws of human energy so that we can manage it better and avoid losing it through ignorance.

As the ancient Egyptians once did to their pharaohs, I wish you life, strength, and health!

BIBLIOGRAPHY

Laure Goldbright

- *Colon Cleansing and Its Benefits for Health and Skin: A Testimonial*

- *Menopause Free of Suffering: A Testimonial*

Arnold Ehret *(www.arnoldeheret.it)*

-*Mucusless Diet Healing System: Scientific Method of Eating Your Way to Health*

- *Rational Fasting, Regeneration Diet and Natural Cure for all Diseases*

- *The Cause and Cure of Human Illness*

- *The Story of My Life*

- *Definite Cure of Chronic Constipation Also Overcoming Constipation Naturally*

- *Thus Speaketh the Stomach (Also the Tragedy of Nutrition)*

Marcel Violet

https://fr.wikipedia.org/wiki/Marcel_Violet

Le Secret des patriarches - Essai sur la nature de l'énergie biologique

Masaru Emoto

- The Hidden Messages in Water
- The Healing Power of Water
- The Miracle of Water
- The True Power of Water: Healing and Discovering Ourselves
- Water Crystal Healing: Music and Images to restore Your Well-being
- Love Thyself: The Message from Water
- Messages from Water and the Universe
- The Shape of Love: Discovering Who We Are, Where We Came From, and Where We're Going

Jacques Benveniste

Ma Vérité sur la « Mémoire de l'eau »

Edmond Bordeaux Szekely

Introduzione alla Cosmoterapia

Christian Tal Schaller e Johanne Razanamahay

- Il Manuale delle Emozioni, Come sconfiggere gli stati mentali che soffocano la tua vita

- Amaroli, l'acqua di vita, Una straordinaria terapia naturale sperimentata con successo da millenni

Michel Moine e Jean-Louis Degaudenzi

Guide de géobiologie: comment vous débarrasser des ondes nocives et des maladies difficiles à soigner

Hulda Clark

- *The Cure for All Diseases: With Many Cases Histories*
- *The Cure for All Advanced Cancers*

Eberhart, N.M. (1920)

A Working Manual of High Frequency Currents, Chicago, IL: New Medicine Publishing Co., pp. 319

Enza Ciccolo

Acqua d'Amore, Terapeutica fonte di vita

L'Energie delle Acque a Luce Bianca, Nell'acqua il dono per rinascere

Kathleen McAuliffe

- *This Is Your Brain on Parasites: How Tiny Creatures Manipulate Our Behavior and Shape Society*

Andreas Ludwig Kalcker

- *Forbidden Health: Incurable Was Yesterday*

Jim Humble and Cari Lloyd

- *MMS Health Recovery Guide Book*

Georges Lakhovsky

- *The Secret of Life: Cosmic Rays and Radiations of Living Beings*
- *Science and Happiness*

Edward Bach

- *The Twelve Healers and other Remedies*
- *Heal Thyself*

OTHER BOOKS IN ENGLISH BY ANNA MANCINI (www.amancini.com)

They are published by Buenos Books America, and available on Amazon and www.buenosbooks.us

-The Meaning of Dreams

-Your Dreams Can Save Your Life: How and Why Yours Dreams Warn You of Every Danger: Tidal Waves, Tornadoes, Storms, Landslides, Plane Crashes, Assaults, Attacks, Burglaries, Etc.

- Your Dreams Can Save Your Health: Signs of Infectious Diseases in Dreams, Dreaming the Right Remedies, Accurate Diagnosis, and Early Detection of Diseases

-Depression and How your Dreams Can Help You Avoid It

-The Clairvoyance of Dreams: What clairvoyance is and how you can simply use your dreams to achieve it

-Tricks to Remember your Dreams

-*Tricks to Sleep Better*

-*Maat revealed, philosophy of justice in ancient Egypt*

-*How to unlock the secrets, enigmas and mysteries of Ancient Egypt and other old civilizations*

-*Internet Justice, philosophy of law for the virtual world*

-*Copyright law is obsolete*

-*International patent law is obsolete*

-*Scientific creativity*

- *Ancient roman solutions to modern legal issues, the example of patent law*

ABOUT ANNA MANCINI

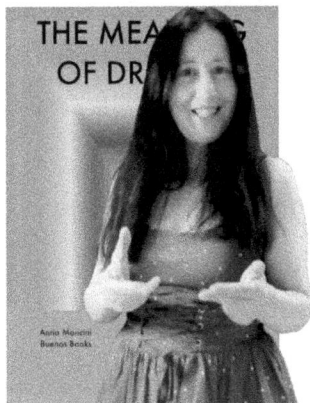

www.amancini.com

Inspired by her family culture, Anna Mancini has been interested in dreams from a young age.

Later, while she was writing her PhD thesis on patent law, a great dream changed her life. This special and very clear dream gave her the solution to a mystery of ancient Roman law that many researchers all over the world had not managed to solve.

For many years she has observed dreams and also dreamers, and has done experiments in order to understand what influence their environment and lifestyle have on the content of their dreams. For her research, she has also made use of old unknown teachings on the human psyche that have survived through the remains of old legal systems.

Thanks to this original method of working on dreams and with the help of her own dreams that have guided her throughout her research, she has been able to:

- develop an innovative and efficient method for the interpretation of oneiric language;

- develop a technique that allows us to ask our subconscious questions and receive answers, whatever the subject area;

- understand which conditions are favorable and unfavorable for creative dreams;

- and discover many other things that make our waking life easier and increase the vitality of dreamers.

She created the research organization 'Innovative You' in 1995, based in Paris, within which she has been able with others to experiment with the techniques for working on dreams that she has developed after long personal research.

She runs workshops, gives lectures and coaches people so that they too can use their dreams to improve all aspects of their lives and also become more creative. She teaches these oneiric creativity techniques in France and abroad, in particular in the research and innovation departments of companies.

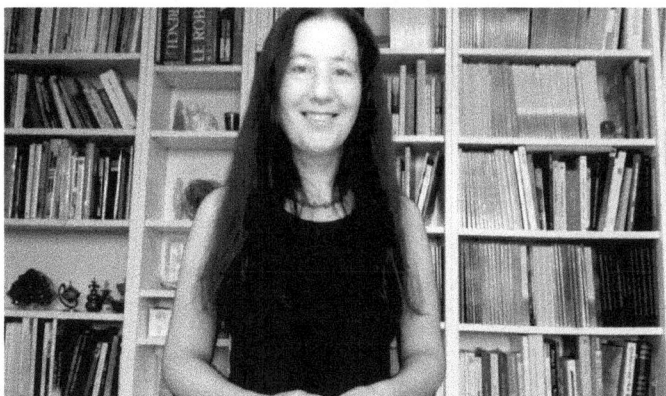

www.amancini.com

CONTENTS